AVERY'S NUTRITION DISCOVERY SERIES

D-RIBOSE

WHAT YOU NEED TO KNOW

EDMUND R. BURKE, Ph.D.

AVERY PUBLISHING GROUP
Garden City Park • New York

The information contained in this book is based upon the research and personal and professional experiences of the author. It is not intended as a substitute for consulting with your physician or other health care provider. Any attempt to diagnose and treat an illness should be done under the direction of a health care professional.

The publisher does not advocate the use of any particular health care protocol, but believes the information in this book should be available to the public. The publisher and author are not responsible for any adverse effects or consequences resulting from the use of any of the suggestions, preparations, or procedures discussed in this book. Should the reader have any questions concerning the appropriateness of any procedure or preparation mentioned, the author and the publisher strongly suggest consulting a professional health care advisor.

Series Cover Designer: Doug Brooks
Cover Image Courtesy of PhotoDisc

Avery Publishing Group, Inc
120 Old Broadway
Garden City Park, NY 11040
1-800-548-5757
or visit us on the web at www.averypublishing.com

Copyright © 1999 by Edmund R. Burke, PhD

ISBN: 0-89529-981-X

All rights reserved. No part of this publication may be reproduced, stored in a retrieval system, or transmitted, in any form or by any means, electronic, mechanical, photocopying, recording, or otherwise, without the prior written consent of the copyright owner.

Printed in the United States of America

10 9 8 7 6 5 4 3 2 1

CONTENTS

Introduction, 1

1. ATP: The Body's Energy Regulator, 3
2. Ribose: What Is This Incredible Nutrient? 7
3. Muscles, Exercise, and Energy, 10
4. Losing Nucleotides During Exercise and Poor Circulation, 15
5. How Ribose Works, 19
6. The Scientific Research, 24
7. Using Ribose, 31

Conclusion, 35

Glossary, 36

Selected References, 39

Index, 42

INTRODUCTION

Your body must be continuously supplied with energy to perform its many complex functions. As the body's energy demands increase with exercise, work, or in various disease states, there must be a way to provide this additional energy or you stop functioning at your optimum level.

The energy-rich chemical compound that provides virtually all the energy needed by your body is known as adenosine triphosphate, or simply ATP. The energy released from the breakdown of ATP is used to power all body functions. We need ATP to make our hearts beat, to give our muscles power when we demand it, and to maintain our everyday lives. Without adequate ATP stores, we could not walk, run, breathe, or even have blood flow through our bodies. So, ATP is considered the "energy currency" of the cell. It is, in fact, the molecule that gives us life.

In normal conditions at rest, our bodies are able to produce all the ATP we need for a healthy existence. However, in stressful conditions, such as doing strenuous high-intensity exercise or when suffering from various diseases, ATP cannot be replaced fast enough. In fact, when ATP is broken down for energy under these conditions, some of the molecules used by the cell to recycle ATP are washed out of the cell and cannot be easily replaced. When that happens, there are not enough of these compounds available to replace ATP as it is used. The result is that cell function, and in fact the continued life of the cell, can be compromised.

To stay healthy and active, to keep our hearts functioning properly and to maintain peak levels of muscle performance, we need to keep this pool of ATP at the highest level possible. This pool of ATP is absolutely vital for our heart and skeletal muscles to have all the energy they need to provide maximum strength and endurance.

Researchers have learned that a simple sugar—D-ribose, also called "ribose"—stimulates the body's production of ATP. In fact, ribose is the essential compound required to make ATP molecules and maintain high levels of energy in the heart and skeletal muscles. If you are young or old, healthy or not, a serious athletic competitor, a weekend athlete, or simply concerned about staying healthy, you should understand the role of ATP in your body and its contribution to your health, fitness, and well being. What does it do? Why do you need it? And most importantly, how does ribose help in maintaining adequate and healthy levels of the total ATP in your body?

Many people can benefit from ribose supplementation. Regardless of how you live or how active you are, you need enough of these compounds to maintain healthy cells functioning at peak performance. In general, though, those that will benefit most from ribose supplementation are athletes and people with conditions that decrease blood flow and oxygen availability to their hearts or skeletal muscles. Ribose supplementation helps athletes because ribose helps to increase energy in the heart and skeletal muscles and replaces muscle cell energy charge during and after bouts of strenuous exercise. It helps people with conditions that decrease blood flow and oxygen availability to their hearts or skeletal muscles, because it helps replace ATP that is broken down in the cells during even light or moderate exercise. Ribose supplementation is also of benefit to anyone simply interested in healthy daily living. Maintaining normal, physiologically active levels of ATP is vital in controlling energy charge in the heart and muscle cells and in regulating the function of enzymes, electrolyte activity, and other important cell functions.

The benefits of ribose have been researched for several years at leading universities in the United States and Europe. These studies show that ribose really works! Ribose has never been available to consumers before because the cost to manufacture this important nutrient has been too high. Only now, after an economical way has been found to manufacture ribose, is it available commercially as a nutritional supplement. And in *D-Ribose: What You Need to Know,* we'll discuss how this supplement can help you, how you should take it, where you can find it, and much more.

1
ATP: THE BODY'S ENERGY REGULATOR

When you use your muscles you are asking them to perform work. You expect that they will work at peak performance, providing strength, power, and endurance. You ask your heart to pump hard enough to supply the blood flow needed by your body to function normally. In addition, you ask your skeletal muscles to lift, turn, stretch, bend, walk, or run at your command. Without the energy provided by ATP, none of these activities would be possible.

Muscle contraction is actually the chemical conversion of the food you eat into mechanical work, such as pedaling a bike or lifting a weight. For this work to be performed muscle cells require fuel to keep the process going. The cycle must be continually repeated so that the muscle cells do not run out of gas. Fuel must continually be fed to the fire of muscular work or the engine will slow down or stop. The food that we eat serves as that fuel. Food is converted in the body to adenosine triphosphate, or ATP, the molecule used by the cell for its total energy supply. ATP is an adenine nucleotide. It is not really important to understand all the complicated biochemistry. However, it is important to know that without these complex molecules your body would not be able to perform any of the activities of daily life. You could not stand, walk, or even breathe. Your heart would stop beating and brain function would stop. Your basic genetic code would be lost and life as you know it would cease. Clearly, ATP and its byproducts (adenosine diphosphate, or ADP and adenosine monophosphate, or AMP) are absolutely essential for life itself and ribose is absolutely essential for the body to form these life-giving compounds.

HOW THE BODY MAKES ATP FOR ENERGY

ATP is produced in the body through a series of chemical reactions beginning with the food you eat. Carbohydrates, fats, and proteins are digested in the stomach and intestines and taken up by the blood for distribution to all the cells of the body. In fact, some of the simple food molecules, such as glucose, begin digestion in the mouth and are moved into the blood stream very quickly for use by your cells. Many of these food compounds are taken from the blood by your cells to make energy, which is stored in the cell as ATP. Other food molecules are used by the cell to form glycogen, which is kept for future use to make energy when it is needed. The balance of the food you eat is used to form proteins for muscle development and fatty acids, which are stored in the body as fat cells. Fat cells are also important storehouses of energy. Your heart, for example, uses fatty acids as the preferred source of fuel for energy production.

Every cell must form its own ATP. This energy-giving molecule cannot be absorbed from the blood or supplied by other tissues but must be formed inside the cell from the nutrients taken from the blood. When ATP is used for energy, the cell must rebuild the ATP it uses from what is left over, or form new ATP molecules through a series of complicated metabolic processes. The cell can store only a limited amount of ATP, so in periods of stress or strenuous exercise ATP molecules must continually be recycled by the cell to maintain a sufficient amount of energy for continued, normal function.

The "A" in ATP, adenosine, is comprised of one molecule of ribose and one molecule of adenine (hence the name adenine nucleotide). The ATP compound is made up of one molecule of adenosine and three phosphate molecules. Energy is produced when the chemical bond holding the last of the three phosphate molecules to the ATP molecule is broken by various biochemical reactions. (See Figure 1.1.) The breaking of this chemical bond produces a great deal of energy for use by the cell. There are only about 90 grams (a little over three ounces) of ATP in the body. This is enough to provide maximal energy for less than 10 seconds. As a result, the cell must constantly recycle ATP to keep the energy process going.

When ATP splits off this last molecule of phosphate, the remaining compounds are ADP, or adenosine diphosphate, and inorganic phosphate, or Pi, which stays in the cell waiting for a new place to attach. In normal circumstances, this ADP molecule is able to reform quickly producing ATP again for additional energy. When there is a plentiful supply of oxygen in the cell (called aerobic metabolism), this process is rapid and utilizes fuels such as glucose or fatty acids in the metabolic processes attaching Pi to ADP re-forming ATP. When there is not a sufficient amount of oxygen present (called anaerobic metabolism), the cell generally uses creatine phosphate

(CrP) as the source of a phosphate molecule for reforming ATP from ADP. Creatine phosphate stores the phosphate molecule in the cell, making it available for use when called upon during stress or heavy exercise.

Even though skeletal muscle cells contain three or four times more creatine phosphate than ATP, they also use their creatine phosphate pools very quickly during intense exercise. In fact, all of the available creatine phosphate in the muscle cell can be used up in only a few seconds of maximal muscular work. In the heart, if there is not enough blood flow to provide the necessary oxygen for normal energy metabolism (called oxidative stress or anoxia), CrP is also used quickly as the cell rebuilds ATP to allow the heart to keep beating.

The Myokinase Reaction

As creatine phosphate pools are used, the muscle cell calls upon yet another metabolic reaction known as the myokinase reaction. The myokinase reaction is a very important reaction used by our skeletal muscle cells to help restore ATP lost during intense exercise. In the myokinase reaction, two molecules of ADP are used to form one molecule of ATP and one molecule of AMP. As the names suggest, adenosine diphosphate (ADP) contains one molecule of adenosine and two molecules of phosphate, while adenosine monophosphate (AMP) contains adenosine and only one molecule of phosphate. The myokinase reaction is an extremely important reaction in skeletal muscle cells. This reaction helps restore energy to the muscle cell while it is under the stress of prolonged, hard work. It also works to keep a balance between ATP and ADP concentrations in the cell. A careful balance of these compounds is necessary to keep the muscle cell working smoothly. If this balance is disturbed, the cell will stop functioning until the balance is restored.

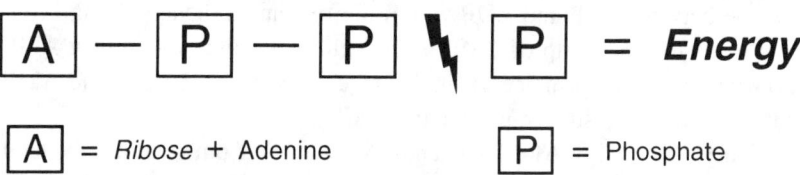

Figure 1.1. ATP molecule creating energy.
When the last phosphate molecule is broken off from the ATP molecule, energy is created.

When the cell has used up its other resources, it turns to the myokinase reaction to restore required energy. The myokinase reaction efficiently rebuilds ATP, but it leads to a build up of AMP in the cell. This build up of AMP can cause problems for the cell, so other reactions are put to use to rid the cell of this extra AMP. Some of the AMP built up in the cell is broken down and pushed out to be lost forever. For the cell to rebuild its total pool of ATP, ADP, and AMP new molecules must be formed. These reactions lead to an ultimate decrease in the total pool of ATP, ADP, and AMP, eventually leaving only a few ATP molecules—not enough for the competitive athlete's energy needs, or any person's prolonged and strenuous activity.

Your body is an exquisitely formed machine. Muscle cells have developed these various metabolic reactions so that during periods of strenuous high-intensity activity or oxidative stress, heart and skeletal muscle cells can maintain adequate levels of energy to perform their required work. Muscle cells use these very intricate reactions to synthesize and conserve as much ATP as possible. However, these cells must also maintain ratios of ATP, ADP, and AMP within very close tolerances. They cannot build up extra pools of one of these molecules at the expense of another. If they are not able to maintain these balances the cell will shut down, losing power, endurance and, in the worst case, causing cell death.

IN SUMMARY

To summarize this process, the net result of these energy-conserving reactions is that during heavy, intense exercise, or periods of oxidative stress, heart and skeletal muscle cells use ATP for energy and other metabolic processes. Because they are not able to recycle ATP at a sufficient rate to replace what they use (called ATP turnover or recycling of ATP), CrP is used as a source of phosphate to recycle ADP to ATP. However, CrP pools are used up quickly in muscle cells, so as a backup system ADP is used (in the myokinase reaction) to assist in rebuilding ATP levels and keeping the balance between ATP and ADP within the tolerances dictated by the cell. This leads to a build up of AMP in the cell, and causes removal of AMP from the cell to help maintain the balance between ATP, ADP, and AMP that is necessary to sustain muscular work.

Large amounts of ATP, ADP, and AMP are lost from heart and skeletal muscle cells during periods of intense exercise or oxidative stress. Ribose is an essential tool used by the body to replace these energy compounds as they are used. Without ribose they cannot be saved or replaced. And, as we will see later, waiting for the body to produce the ribose needed to rebuild these molecules takes a great deal of time and affects function of the muscle cell.

2

RIBOSE: WHAT IS THIS INCREDIBLE NUTRIENT?

Ribose (pronounced rye'-bose) is a simple sugar that is extremely important in many processes in your body. Metabolism of ribose was first researched in the 1930s, but it was not until the 1950s that the importance of ribose truly began to be known. Until that time, the techniques of biochemical research were not adequate to determine the very complicated processes that use ribose in the body. However, since that time, a large volume of research has been done looking at the many roles played by ribose in metabolism. Beginning in the 1970s ribose began to be recognized as an important compound in treating poor circulation in the heart and by the 1980s this research was actively pursued by scientists. Research throughout the 1980s and early 1990s showed conclusively that giving ribose to people suffering from poor blood flow increased the energy level in their hearts by a wide margin. It wasn't until the early 1990s that a similar result was found in skeletal muscle.

RIBOSE: A NATURAL SUGAR

Ribose is a sugar. It is, then, a carbohydrate. The carbohydrate backbone of ribonucleic acid (RNA) and a cell's genes, deoxyribonucleic acid (DNA), is ribose and deoxyribose, respectively. These nucleic acids contain the information necessary for cells to grow, develop, divide, and carry out their normal functions. They are also the genetic materials used to pass on the genetic code from one generation to the next.

Ribose is found in all living cells. In addition to being the backbone of genetic material, ribose is also the starting point for production of ATP, which is the only molecule your body uses for energy. Your cells cannot function or survive without energy, and energy cannot be produced without ribose to make ATP and other adenine nucleotides. As you will see, high-intensity exercise and certain metabolic or medical conditions cause your body to lose these critical energy-producing molecules. Ribose is the only supplement available that helps your heart and muscle cells restore these life-giving compounds when they are lost and need to be replaced.

When you exercise, some of the ATP that is used for energy is lost from the cell and must be replaced. Ribose is the only compound the body uses as a starting point to replace these energy-producing molecules. Ribose production in the heart and skeletal muscles, however, is a slow process that cannot keep up with this loss of energy when you suffer from ischemia (poor blood flow to the heart or other organ) or during strenuous, intense exercise. Under normal conditions, it may take several days to completely replace the energy molecules that are lost due to ischemia or heavy exercise.

While all living cells contain ribose, there is not enough in food to provide the beneficial effects needed to keep energy levels high during strenuous exercise or ischemia. Ribose in meat is predominately lost by cooking. In fact, ribose reacting with amino acids in the protein causes the chemical process in meat that turns it brown and gives it the characteristic aroma and flavor when it is cooked. Ribose in plant foodstuffs is insufficient to provide meaningful levels to the body.

While it is not important to understand how the body produces ribose, you should know that supplemental ribose bypasses the slow, rate-limiting steps the body uses to make this substance from glucose. Supplemental ribose is able to go directly to work at rebuilding energy-producing molecules as the cell uses them. As a result, your body is able to rebuild its energy supply quickly, making it available to restore peak performance.

RIBOSE ... THE SUPREME ENERGY SOURCE

Ribose is used by the body in three ways. The first is in the manufacture of glucose. Glucose is the simple sugar used by the body to perform many basic metabolic activities. For example, it is used for many of the metabolic processes required for energy production and is a key starting point for many other necessary cellular functions—including, in turn, producing ribose. Second, ribose may be converted to form pyruvate, which enters the metabolic pathways leading to ATP production in the presence of oxygen supplied by the blood stream. Third, ribose is the key compound used by the body to form nucleotides. This is the most important role played by ribose. In this role, ribose helps maintain an adequate pool of these necessary compounds in heart, skeletal muscle, and other cells of the body. Ribose is absolutely essential for the body to produce these life-giving nucleotides. Nucleotides, in turn, are essential compounds required by the body to perform the following functions:

- Produce energy required by muscle cells for strength, endurance, and performance and to fuel all the metabolic reactions necessary for life itself.
- Manufacture protein, glycogen, and nucleic acids (RNA and DNA), all of which are required by the body for normal function.
- Form compounds called cyclic nucleotides that are necessary for controlling the activity of calcium and other electrolytes in the cell. The most important controlling function performed by these compounds is assisting in contraction and relaxation of heart and muscle cells. Nucleotides are also required to control the enzymes necessary to regulate electrolyte levels in muscle cells.
- Transfer energy from one compound to the next. The cell requires this energy transfer to fuel normal activity.

Ribose is also used by pharmaceutical companies to manufacture many compounds that are important to our health. Riboflavin, one of the essential B-complex vitamins, is made from ribose. Many drugs also use ribose as a key ingredient. Anti-viral drugs, for example, use ribose as important parts of their chemical structure.

Although ribose is found naturally in all the cells in the body, heart and skeletal muscle cannot make ribose very quickly. In fact, during times of metabolic stress, such as during strenuous exercise or diminished blood flow, your cells are not able to form enough ribose to rapidly replace nucleotides as they are used. Furthermore, there is no known food source that supplies a sufficient amount of ribose to be metabolically significant. Therefore, ribose supplementation is essential to quickly replace ATP, ADP, and AMP as they are used by the cell.

Describing the actual way ribose works in heart and skeletal muscle cells is the main topic of this booklet. However, it is a complicated process that cannot be described in a few words. In fact, to get a better understanding of the role of ribose in metabolism, you first must understand how the body manages its energy production and metabolism in muscle and heart cells. This basic understanding is essential in truly appreciating the significant role ribose plays in our lives every day.

3

MUSCLES, EXERCISE, AND ENERGY

Muscles are the machines we use to perform work. We all know that without muscles we could not stand, lift, run, turn, or jump. What we may not know, though, is that muscles perform many other necessary functions. The heart is a muscle, and without a fit heart we could not pump enough blood to keep all of the other machinery in the body going. The diaphragm is a muscle, and without its help we could not breathe. Blood vessels are also muscles, and if they are stiff or clogged we cannot get enough blood through them to provide our cells with energy. Keeping our muscles fit, healthy, and in peak shape is absolutely vital. And, all muscles require a constant supply of energy for peak performance.

TYPES OF MUSCLE

Your body contains two basic types of muscle. The first group is called *smooth* or involuntary muscle, some of which are the blood vessels, the diaphragm, and other muscles that are not made up of long strings of fibers. These muscles function without voluntary thought. Your blood flows through veins and arteries that expand and contract without our mental input. You breathe, forcing your diaphragm to contract and relax without conscious effort. Little research is available that looks at energy production in these muscles or the importance of energy regulation in them. However, you can be sure that these muscles require constant and secure energy supplies, just as your other muscles do. They also require stable pools of ATP to maintain healthy, normal function.

The heart and skeletal muscles, on the other hand, are known as *striated* muscles because they are made up of long strands of muscle fibers. Most striated muscles are also known as voluntary muscles, because they permit voluntary motion at your urging. The heart, of course, is striated but not voluntary. It beats regularly without your conscious effort. Furthermore, there are other differences in heart muscle, so it will be treated separately here. These striated muscles are most important in our discussion. They are the muscles used to provide strength, to perform work and maintain our normal activities.

There are over 430 voluntary muscles in the human body. You call upon these muscles every day for normal living. Each of these muscles performs a specific function. Muscles are made up mostly of water and protein. In fact, about 75 percent of their mass is water, another 20 percent is protein, and the remaining 5 percent is made up of smaller amounts of various substances, including minerals, enzymes, and ribose. You ask these muscles to perform for you in many different situations. In turn, you need to keep them in peak condition. Ribose can help you do that.

Skeletal Muscles

Skeletal muscles are comprised of two different types of muscle fibers, fast-twitch (FT) and slow-twitch (ST). Everyone has both types of muscle fibers in their skeletal muscles, however the amount of each fiber type any individual person may have varies widely. Some athletes, for example, have eight or nine times as many FT fibers in their muscles than ST, but generally, people have about the same number of each. The ratio of FT to ST fibers are thought to be controlled genetically and no amount of training can alter the make up of fibers in the muscle. All fiber types, however, respond to training by improving their ability to perform.

Research has shown that taking ribose has a positive effect on ATP production in all of these muscle fiber types. We will look at specifics more closely later on, but in general it has been found that giving ribose increases the manufacture of ATP in skeletal muscle by 340 percent to 430 percent. It is also reported that ribose improves the cells' ability to salvage and reuse ADP and AMP by as much as 700 percent. These are incredible statistics!

Fast-Twitch Muscle Fibers

As the name implies, fast-twitch (FT) fibers respond rapidly when called upon for contraction. During moderate- to high-intensity exercise they produce brief but powerful contractions because they are able to release calcium quickly, leading to rapid contractions. These FT fibers are used almost exclusively in athletic performance requiring sudden, powerful outbursts, such as sprinting, weightlifting, and playing football. They are also called upon for stop-and-go activities, like those found in basketball, volleyball, and soccer that require sudden spurts of high-energy performance.

Because FT contractions are rapid and powerful, FT fibers use their ATP pools quickly. Much of their work is done under anaerobic conditions because these fibers generally cannot get enough oxygen from the blood to fuel aerobic metabolism during periods of peak supramaximal activity. As such, in these cells creatine phosphate (CrP) is called upon to rapidly phosphorylate ADP in the mitochondria. As this pool is reduced, the compounds making up the AMP are lost from the cell and cannot be used again to further rebuild ATP. However, pools of CrP are not adequate to maintain prolonged contraction. Therefore, in FT fibers the myokinase reaction (discussed in the last chapter) is important to maintain ATP levels, prolong vigorous contraction, and control the ratio of ATP to ADP in the cell. You will recall that the myokinase reaction leads to a build up of AMP in the cell, and the cell needs to reduce this pool of AMP to maintain normal, active function.

Ribose is the compound used by the cell to begin the process of replacing these compounds. Ribose can also slow the rate at which these molecules are lost. As a result, ribose helps cells save, restore, and rebuild energy in working muscle cells.

Slow-Twitch Muscle Fibers

Slow-twitch (ST) muscle fibers are used when a slower speed of contraction is required, such as in bicycle touring, jogging, and walking. Because of their slower response, they are best suited to less intensive aerobic activities and are, therefore, less susceptible to fatigue. Slow-twitch fibers have a high capacity to produce ATP in conditions where oxygen is available. Generally these fibers have greater blood flow supplying more oxygen and have a greater number of mitochondria available to manufacture ATP. (Mitochondria are the furnaces in the cell that convert the food fuel into the fire of energy.)

During exercise, then, both FT and ST fibers use ATP and form chemical products that can move quickly out of the cell called *substrate molecules*. Loss of these substrate molecules causes a significant decrease in energy availability. To return the muscle cells to peak levels of energy, and to maintain high level of performance, these substrate molecules must be replaced. Ribose helps the cell rapidly replace these energy giving compounds.

Heart Muscle

The heart is set apart from all other types of muscle. Heart muscle has a greater ability to use oxygen for ATP regeneration than any other muscle fiber type and, in fact, has almost no capacity for anaerobic metabolism. As such, the heart muscle requires an almost continual supply of oxygen to perform. Under normal conditions, the heart works very well by taking in as much oxygen as it needs for contraction and energy recycling. In fact, blood flow to the heart is preferentially increased as the heart muscle cells call for more energy. When the heart needs blood flow, our bodies direct blood from other parts of the body and send it to the heart to provide additional oxygen. When there is a sufficient amount of oxygen present the heart recycles almost all of its ATP as it is used for energy.

However, when blood flow to the heart is restricted, there is not enough oxygen supply and the muscle cells are not able to keep up with this ATP recycling process. The condition in which blood flow to an organ is decreased is called *ischemia*. Ischemia occurs in the heart when blood flow is restricted, such as in coronary artery disease (or clogged arteries) or when oxygen demands by the heart are not met by blood flow. Sometimes, as is the case with open-heart surgery, ischemia is caused on purpose. Blood flow to the heart is stopped and oxygen is supplied to the body by having a machine put oxygen into the blood and take carbon dioxide out. This process is called cardiopulmonary bypass and it is used whenever the heart is stopped for surgery. In most cases, however, ischemia is caused by heart conditions or ailments that restrict blood flow to the heart muscle. It can also be caused in periods of strenuous exercise that go beyond the ability of the heart to absorb the required amount of oxygen from the blood. This condition is called anoxia.

No matter the cause, during ischemia or anoxia ATP is degraded beyond the ability of the heart to recycle new ATP molecules. Consequently, AMP build-up occurs. Because the heart has almost no capacity to conserve nucleotides, almost the entire amount of AMP formed is rapidly degraded and lost.

Ischemia and anoxia are conditions that can also occur in organs other than the heart. Skeletal muscle can also suffer from both ischemia and anoxia. Some disease states, such as peripheral vascular disease or diabetes, restrict blood flow to skeletal muscles also creating an ischemic condition. In these situations, the cells may not react normally and metabolic conditions similar to those found in heart cells may occur. Loss of ATP, ADP, and AMP from the cells in these conditions may be very significant.

Severe pain, cramping, stiffness, and soreness may result. In severe cases people suffering from these conditions may not be able to perform even the most basic physical activities.

Similarly, there are certain enzyme disorders that cause muscle cells to lose nucleotides. Myoadenylate deaminase deficiency (MADD), for example, is a disorder in which the skeletal muscles are not able to conserve nucleotides. When this happens, AMP formed by the cells is quickly degraded to compounds that cannot be retained by the cell and are lost. Again, pain, cramping, and soreness may result and may last for several days while the muscle cells rebuild energy. It has been reported, in fact, that people suffering from MADD may not even be able to walk across a room without muscle pain. This shows how quickly the loss of nucleotides by the cell can affect muscle function.

In the next chapter we will examine the normal loss of these nucleotides in muscles.

4

LOSING NUCLEOTIDES DURING EXERCISE AND POOR CIRCULATION

Although our heart and muscle cells have evolved very elaborate mechanisms to form, recycle, and conserve energy-producing molecules, they are not always successful in keeping sufficient levels of ATP, ADP, and AMP available. Intense exercise or ischemia (insufficient blood flow) may cause significant loss of nucleotides that leave the cell starving for energy. Obviously, when this happens the function of the cell may be at risk. Weightlifters may not be able to generate the powerful contractions they demand, and the weight they were able to lift only a day or two ago may be impossible to move. Your heart may not pump enough blood to supply your tissues with adequate amounts of oxygen.

Under conditions of maximal exercise, there is a substantial decrease in the total ATP, ADP, and AMP pools in skeletal muscle cells. In fact, research has shown that decreases in these nucleotides can be as much as 20 percent to 28 percent after periods of high-intensity exercise. Both fast-twitch and slow-twitch muscle fibers use ATP to provide energy for contraction. During strenuous exercise, ATP is broken down, rapidly causing AMP to build up in the cell. Some, but not all, of the AMP formed by either FT or ST fibers can be converted to other compounds that give the cell the ability to conserve energy-producing molecules to continue to fuel its work. A substantial portion of the AMP, however, is broken down and washed out of the cell. It is this breakdown of AMP, and the loss of breakdown products, that depletes the cell of its energy-producing compounds.

HOW MUCH ATP IS LOST FROM EXERCISE?

Is the amount of ATP, ADP, and AMP loss during exercise really significant? The simple answer to that question is, yes! Skeletal muscles are very efficient at conserving energy. However, when they are called upon to perform maximum work, the number of energy-producing or energy-conserving molecules that are lost can be significant. As long as there is a sufficient amount of oxygen present in the cell for aerobic metabolism, muscle cells are able to recycle energy virtually without losing any adenine nucleotides. Nevertheless, during periods of very hard supramaximal work, when there is not enough oxygen absorbed into the blood stream to supply the demand of the cells, a large percentage of the total pool of ATP, ADP, and AMP can be lost.

A considerable amount of research has been done to show that the loss of adenine nucleotides by skeletal muscle can be severe during periods of intense exercise or ischemia. One very important study was performed at the Karolinska Institute in Stockholm, Sweden, which is one of the foremost centers for skeletal muscle research in the world. In this study, 11 healthy male volunteers underwent six weeks of high-intensity training three times per week, followed by one week with two training sessions per day. A second group of 9 healthy volunteers rested for the first six weeks, but trained twice a day along with the first group during the final week. A small amount of muscle tissue was taken from the thigh of each of the subjects to analyze the amount of adenine nucleotides present following these periods of exercise and for three days following the final day of training. Muscle tissue samples were also taken before exercise began as a point of comparison.

This research showed that ATP levels in the thigh muscles of the first group dropped 13 percent during the six weeks of training. ATP levels in the muscle tissues of this group did not go down further during the final week of training. This shows that after a period of intense exercise ATP, ADP, and AMP all dropped to well below pre-training levels. More significant, however, is the fact that even after three days of rest following the last exercise bout, ATP levels in this first group still did not recover to pre-training levels. In fact, ATP in the muscle cells of these subjects were still almost 10 percent below their pre-training levels. In other words, even after this three-day rest period the thigh muscles were not able to fully replace their lost ATP.

In the second group, the effect was even more dramatic! This group did not have a period of training before beginning high-intensity exercise in the final week. In fact, they went from being sedentary to performing two exercise bouts per day for one week. In this group, ATP in thigh muscle dropped by 25 percent immediately after the last exercise bout. Even after three days of rest, this group still had an ATP pool that was 19.5 percent less than it had initially! Think of it. The total energy currency in the thigh muscles of this group dropped by 25 percent after intense exercise, and was still almost 20 percent lower than normal even after three days of rest!

These dramatic results show that energy-producing compounds are lost from the cell during exercise and do not recover even after three days of rest. In their paper these researchers concluded, "... repeated high-intensity intermittent exercise caused a decrease in resting levels of skeletal muscle adenine nucleotides [ATP]....The decrease was greater when exercise was more frequently repeated."

In a similar study, Dr. Stathis, at Victoria University in Australia, worked with other researchers to show that thigh muscle ATP levels fell by 19 percent after seven weeks of sprint training. These researchers concluded, "We observed reductions in resting ATP [and TAN, or total adenine nucleotides] after training and attribute these primarily to the inability of muscle to completely restore the purine base lost as a result of high ATP turnover rates during training sessions." In other words, because of exercise, these muscle cells lost the molecules necessary to recharge their energy.

HOW DOES POOR CIRCULATION CAUSE LOSS OF ENERGY IN THE HEART?

Maintaining a healthy heart means that we have to be aware of its needs. Among those needs is maintenance of adequate energy supplies to allow the heart to perform normally. When the heart is starved of energy, it is not able to perform its work properly. Energy is required for the contraction, or pumping, that provides blood flow to the body. Surprisingly, maximal levels of ATP are also required for relaxation. If the heart is not allowed to relax properly, it cannot fill with enough blood and the total blood flow through the heart is decreased.

Heart cells show even higher losses of energy charge during ischemia than skeletal muscles. In one study done at the University of Minnesota, researchers showed that 15 minutes of ischemia in the heart led to a decrease in ATP by an amount greater than 50 percent! This study was done in dogs and was performed to mimic the effect of stopping the heart during surgery. Previous research has shown that the action of ATP metabolism in dogs and other animals is similar to that in man, so the comparison is a good one. In the University of Minnesota study, ATP and total energy charge did not recover even 24 hours after blood flow was returned to the heart. It was reported in this study that it takes 7 to 10 days for ATP levels to fully recover following severe ischemia.

And these study results are reinforced by similar results of many other studies. In 1984, Dr. Heinz-Gerd Zimmer, who is now the head of the physiology department at the Carl-Ludwig Institute at the University of Leipzig, Germany, reported a similar finding. In his study, temporary ischemia of 15 minutes caused about a 45 percent decrease in ATP content. He showed that ATP recovered a slight amount immediately after ischemia as the AMP content of the cell attached to additional phosphate groups to recycle ATP. However, even after three days, ATP levels in the heart did not recover to the levels that were present before ischemia occurred. In another study, Dr. Herbert Ward and his associates showed that even after 48 hours of full blood flow following ischemia ATP levels only recovered to 53 percent of pre-ischemic levels.

HOW CAN YOU PREVENT THE ENERGY LOSS?

The bottom line is this. No matter how hard you try to stop it, no matter what foods you eat or supplements you take (except ribose), if you are actively exercising, then you are losing the compounds necessary to maintain maximum levels of energy in your muscle cells. If you have poor circulation to your heart or other muscles, a metabolic imbalance or a muscle cell enzyme deficiency, you are losing energy compounds. Certain things may be done to reduce the number of these compounds lost from your cells, but in the end, if you are using your muscles for strenuous, high-intensity exercise your energy pools will decrease. The best you can hope for is rapid replacement of lost energy-producing compounds so that your muscle cell energy charge can return to its peak efficiency. As we will see in the following chapters, ribose is essential in the metabolic processes used by the heart and skeletal muscles to recycle and replace these compounds as they are used up or lost.

5

HOW RIBOSE WORKS

It is clear that a large amount of ATP, ADP, and AMP can be lost from both heart and skeletal muscle cells during strenuous exercise or poor circulation. It is equally clear that maximal levels of these compounds are necessary to provide the energy required for peak muscle cell efficiency. Finally, it is unfortunately clear that replacement of these nucleotide pools takes a long time. In skeletal muscles, they may not be replaced even after three days of rest. In the heart, it may take up to 10 days! In this chapter we will examine how these cells replace these lost energy molecules and why it takes so long.

REPLACING LOST ENERGY

Ribose is an essential ingredient in the formation and conservation of ATP, ADP, and AMP. Our heart and skeletal muscles are very elaborate, intricate, and complicated pieces of metabolic machinery that have developed two methods for either building or conserving nucleotides in heart and skeletal muscle cells. Both of these metabolic routes center on ribose as the key compound for energy recovery.

The two metabolic routes for energy recovery are appropriately named. The *salvage* pathway assists the cell in keeping, or salvaging, the end products of AMP breakdown. These end products are lost from the cell quickly if there is not enough ribose in the cell to keep, or salvage, them. In the salvage pathway, it is possible to trap these metabolic products before they leave the cell. When this happens, the products from the breakdown of AMP can be recycled back to AMP. AMP, of course, can then be reconverted to ATP to recharge the cell's energy level.

Obviously, if these metabolic end products have left the cell they cannot be salvaged. When this happens, the muscle cell is forced to manufacture new energy-producing molecules to rebuild the energy charge of the cell. The metabolic routes followed by muscle cells to form new compounds are called *de novo* metabolic pathways. *De novo* is a Latin term meaning *new*. As might be expected, the *de novo* pathways are slower than the salvage pathways since in the salvage pathways the basic compounds are already there. During *de novo* synthesis, however, these compounds are made from scratch beginning with ribose.

Ribose is absolutely essential for either salvage or *de novo* synthetic reactions to work. To begin either the process of salvage or *de novo* synthesis, ribose is converted to a fairly simple molecule with a very complicated name, 5-phosphoribosyl-1-pyrophosphate (generally called PRPP). Energy-producing compounds cannot be salvaged or manufactured by the cell without this molecule. PRPP is formed naturally by the cell. Ribose is immediately converted by the cell to PRPP whenever PRPP is needed. However, the pool of PRPP is limited. During strenuous exercise or in conditions of poor circulation, PRPP may be used up as the cell tries to salvage energy-producing compounds before they are lost from the cell. If there is not a sufficient amount of ribose available to recharge the PRPP pool, muscle cells are not able to save or re-manufacture these compounds.

Again, the bottom line is this. The more ribose you have available for PRPP production, the more of these energy-producing compounds you can salvage and the more ATP you can make. At the same time, if you are serious about your exercise regimen you will lose ATP pools during strenuous, high-intensity training. Having peak levels of ATP allows you to perform at your best—with peak results. Ribose will help in replacing these lost nucleotides quickly. Ribose is absolutely, unequivocally required to conserve energy-producing compounds in the cell or to manufacture new compounds if they are lost. Without ribose, our heart and skeletal muscle cells would not be able to maintain adequate levels of energy to perform their work. The main aim is, therefore, to elevate the restricted PRPP pool and keep it high. This can only be accomplished by administration of ribose.

YOUR BODY JUST CAN'T GET ENOUGH!

If ribose is not taken as a supplement, it must be manufactured by heart and skeletal muscle cells so that energy molecules can be produced and energy charge in the cells can be maintained. To form PRPP without ribose supplementation, glucose must be converted to ribose through a series of complicated chemical reactions. Ribose thus formed is then immediately converted to PRPP. The metabolic pathway used by the body to form ribose is slow and uses even more of the cell's energy. This slow process of forming ribose from glucose may take several days. That is why it takes so long to fully restore energy in the heart and skeletal muscles after exhaustive exercise or ischemia.

The pathway converting glucose to ribose is controlled by one specific enzymatic step. The enzyme that controls this very important process is called glucose-6-phosphate dehydrogenase (G-6-PDH). In both the heart and skeletal muscle, this enzyme is in very short supply. This enzyme ultimately controls the amount of ribose that can be produced in your body. Supplemental ribose bypasses the limiting enzymatic step through G-6-PDH and goes directly to PRPP so that energy can be produced or conserved quickly. Consequently, recovery of ATP both during and following strenuous exercise or ischemia can be dramatically improved.

PRPP formed through ribose supplementation is immediately available to conserve energy in heart and skeletal muscle cells and can quickly manufacture new energy-producing molecules that are lost in strenuous exercise or ischemia.

WHY IS IT NECESSARY TO SUPPLEMENT WITH RIBOSE?

On average, the human body contains 1.6 milligrams (mg) of ribose per 100 milliliters (ml) of blood at any given time. Some people do not have any free ribose in their blood while others have as much as 3.6 mg per 100 ml. There are no foods that provide enough ribose from the diet to be helpful. Of course, since all living cells contain ribose, a small amount is taken in every time we eat. Taking ribose as a dietary supplement is required to rapidly increase the levels of ribose in the blood, making it available to the cells in building up PRPP pools and building energy. When taken as a supplement, ribose is absorbed very quickly into the bloodstream, with much of the absorption occurring before the ribose is even swallowed.

RIBOSE—WHERE HAVE YOU BEEN ALL MY LIFE?

Ribose has been studied for a long time. In 1958 the metabolism of ribose in man was studied showing how ribose is absorbed and used by the body. It was only in the late 1970s that ribose began to be recognized as an important compound in treating circulation problems in the heart. In the late 1970s, through the 1980s, and into the 1990s, hundreds of research papers have been published in respected medical journals in the U.S. and Europe focusing primarily on the effects of ribose in fighting heart disease.

These studies have shown conclusively that exercise and poor circulation lead to decreases in cellular energy pools and energy availability in the heart and skeletal muscle. They have shown further that this decrease in energy charge affects muscle cell function. Research has been conducted in rats, swine, dogs, and humans. All of the research points to the same thing, that supplemental ribose increases ATP levels in the heart and skeletal muscle cells following high-intensity exercise or diminished blood flow and that function can be improved with ribose. Several of these research studies will be discussed in more detail later.

Although researchers have long recognized the benefits of ribose, the cost of manufacturing this important nutrient has been too high to make it commercially available. Only recently has a process been developed to inexpensively produce ribose. That is why it has taken so long for this important compound to be available to consumers.

A CASE STUDY

Darrell Buttshaw is a 67-year-old Minnesotan who was forced to retire early from his job as a food plant supervisor. Darrell, or Bucky as his friends call him, has 99 percent blockage of the left main artery to his heart. He has 100 percent blockage of the right main artery. In 1986, he underwent a triple coronary artery bypass operation. These arteries are now also suffering from blockage. Bucky has always been an active man who likes to walk, play golf, and bowl. His disease, however, has prevented most of these activities since even light exercise causes severe chest pain requiring him to take nitroglycerine tablets. To get some exercise, however, Bucky and his wife would take walks. He could go only a few blocks before chest pain forced him to stop, take a nitroglycerine tablet and rest until the pain went away. However, he would persist with walking, taking nitroglycerine, and resting until he went as far as he thought he should go.

About one year ago, he heard about ribose. He started to take "two heaping teaspoons a day," or about 15 to 20 grams. He generally mixed the ribose in juice or cold water. After about two days he began to notice an effect. He was able to walk farther—in fact, up to two miles—without chest pain. He was able to do things in the yard and he could begin golf and bowling again all without the pain he would otherwise have. When he ran out of ribose, his symptoms of chest pain would return and he would be right back on the nitroglycerine tablets again.

Now, he takes "one heaping teaspoon" a day, or about five to ten grams. He is still able to perform his daily routine, including walking two miles, without chest pain. At a recent consultation with his cardiologist, he was told, "I don't know what you are doing, but keep doing it!" Bucky is a definite believer in the positive effects of ribose!

Of course this is the story of only one person and is not the result of a scientifically administered double blind clinical study. But the improvement in his condition as the result of ribose administration was enough evidence to convince him. It also gives good anecdotal evidence as to the effectiveness of supplemental ribose. But there is some scientific evidence out there to support the effectiveness of ribose, as we shall see in the next chapter.

6
THE SCIENTIFIC RESEARCH

Scientific evidence on ribose is clear. It works to rebuild and restore energy in heart and skeletal muscle cells. Period.

Data on the specific effects of ribose on athletic performance is less clear. There simply is not enough research completed yet to make definitive statements possible. However, research showing the effects of ribose in test animals gives a strong indication that similar positive results should be expected in humans. Unfortunately, there are only a few researchers doing studies on ribose in skeletal muscle. More and more researchers are gaining an appreciation for the effects of ribose, however, and we expect this situation to change in the near future.

RIBOSE AND THE HEART

There has been a great deal of research to show that ribose helps the heart increase its energy and function following periods of poor circulation. When blood flow to the heart muscle itself is decreased, it is not able to get enough oxygen from the blood to maintain normal activity. Many things can cause this lack of circulation to the heart. For example, coronary artery disease can be caused by high cholesterol or triglycerides in the blood and may lead to decreased blood flow through the arteries of the heart. When coronary artery disease exists, the heart may not get enough blood to supply even basic needs. Light activity, such as walking, may be impossible without chest pain. If this condition becomes severe, normal routine activities may be impossible to perform and a heart attack may be the ultimate result. Other things may also restrict circulation to the heart. Sudden strenuous exercise without proper warm up may be a cause. Additionally, heart surgery intentionally stops circulation when the heart is stopped for surgery. Finally, exercising beyond the heart's ability to take up oxygen may cause anoxia, a condition in which the heart does not get enough oxygen to function normally.

Both poor circulation and anoxia significantly decrease the energy charge in the heart. During both of these conditions, ATP levels in the heart may decrease by as much as 50 percent or more. Restoring blood flow has only a marginal affect on increasing the ATP levels. One study showed that after one hour of normal blood flow after it was first restricted, ATP recovered to only 60 percent of the level that was present before the circulation was stopped. In other words, ATP levels were still decreased by 40 percent below normal! This study also determined that this decrease in ATP levels had a negative effect on heart function that was directly related to ATP in the heart. Function did not return to normal until ATP levels increased to their normal values. Interestingly, creatine phosphate levels in the heart returned to normal almost immediately after blood flow was resumed, but did not affect the ability of the heart to rebuild ATP stores. Obviously, the compounds necessary to replace the lost ATP were missing. They had been washed out of the heart during the time that circulation was restricted.

Other research has found similar results. A study done at the University of Minnesota determined that ATP levels fell by 50 percent after circulation was restricted and suggested that it may take 7 to 10 days for ATP levels to return to normal. Giving ribose allowed the heart to recover 85 percent of its ATP within 24 hours. In another study, after the heart was stopped, ATP levels dropped by 48 percent and took 9.9 days to return to normal. Again, giving ribose returned ATP levels to normal within 1.2 days. Researchers at the Max-Plank Institute in Bad Nauheim, Germany found that giving ribose increased the rate of ATP synthesis by 500 percent after blood flow to the heart was cut off. Other German researchers found that ribose increased ATP metabolism by 90 percent during the first 60 minutes of recovery from a restriction in circulation that lasted only 4.5 minutes. Finally, in another German study, it was found that ribose increased the ability of the heart to recover from heart attack. Both ATP levels and heart function returned to normal within two days, but without ribose heart function was still depressed after four weeks.

The studies summarized above all took place in test animals. However, the effects of ribose and ATP recovery have been found to be similar in humans. In research performed at West Virginia University (yet unpublished), Dr. Robert Vance studied the effect of ribose on heart function following surgery. Dr. Vance found that, following surgery, patients who were not given ribose had a decrease of almost 40 percent in the amount of blood that the heart could pump. In patients given ribose, there was no decrease. These hearts maintained their ability to pump adequate blood supply to the body even after their hearts were stopped.

Dr. Wolfgang Pliml conducted a benchmark study at the University of Munich, Germany. In this study, Dr. Pliml looked at patients with severe but stable coronary artery disease. These patients suffered from severe chest pain when they were asked to exercise on a treadmill for short periods of time. In addition, they showed changes in their electrocardiograms (a measure of heart function) during exercise. Dr. Pliml asked these patients to exercise until their heart function changed or until they had severe chest pain. After the preliminary treadmill tests were given, half of the study group was given ribose and the other half was given glucose as a placebo. Each group took the prescribed dose of ribose or placebo for three days and then another treadmill test was given. In this final test, the group given ribose could exercise significantly longer than the placebo (glucose) group before changes occurred in their electrocardiograms. Additionally, the ribose patients were able to exercise much longer after ribose administration than they could before getting ribose.

All of these findings show that ribose has a direct and significant effect on the heart after restricted blood flow or anoxia. But how about before these conditions exist? Should ribose be taken then? The answer is yes! Dr. John Chatham and his associates at Oxford University in England answered this question conclusively. In their study, these researchers showed that giving ribose both before and after blood flow was restricted led to a faster recovery of ATP levels than giving ribose only after the restriction occurred. Giving of ribose after a circulatory problem occurred increased the rate of ATP recovery in the heart dramatically. However, giving ribose both before and after restricted flow allowed the heart to recover its energy charge even more quickly. They concluded that, "Ribose may be functioning in several ways to maintain ATP." This research showed that taking ribose to maintain high levels in the heart before circulatory problems or anoxia occurred improved the heart's ability to keep its energy levels at their peak.

Many, many, such studies exist showing how ribose improves the ability of the heart to increase ATP levels, rebuild total energy charge, and improve function following a decrease in oxygen supply. Ribose taken before, during, and after such circulatory and anoxic events will help the heart maintain the high level of efficiency we demand for maximum performance.

RIBOSE AND SKELETAL MUSCLE

The direct effect of ribose in improving energy charge in skeletal muscle has not been widely studied. However, one researcher, Dr. Ronald Terjung, now at Missouri University, has conducted significant research in this field. Dr. Terjung has researched several aspects of energy metabolism and energy charge in skeletal muscle. In one study performed in his laboratory, it was determined that fast-twitch muscle was able to form energy-saving compounds from AMP as a means to conserve cellular energy. Slow-twitch fibers did not form high levels of these compounds and lost more of the AMP break-down products formed during exercise. Then he found that after intense running, these energy-conserving compounds (in both fast-twitch and slow-twitch muscle) were degraded and the end products were found in the blood. He concluded that when muscle concentrations of these compounds continued to increase during running exercise, they were degraded and lost from the muscle cell into the blood. The net result of this was a decrease in ATP recovery following intense exercise. Ribose may play an important role in recovery of these ATP pools.

In another study, Dr. Terjung and his fellow researchers found that after three minutes of strenuous contractions with constant blood flow (or aerobic contraction), the loss of ATP in slow-twitch muscle fibers was a significant 10 percent. When blood flow was restricted, as would be the case with anaerobic exercise, the results were even more significant. In this case, low levels of contraction for 10 minutes led to a decrease in ATP levels of 47 percent. Additional research in slow-twitch fibers showed that 10 minutes of mild contraction decreased ATP levels by 40 percent. Again, it is clear that exercise decreases the energy charge of muscle cells and that this energy charge must be replaced to restore the muscle to full strength. Ribose can be effective in helping muscles restore the energy charge in muscle cells.

Researchers at the State University of New York at Syracuse, and the Copenhagen Muscle Research Center, Copenhagen, Denmark, conducted research on human subjects. This study showed that during intense, exhaustive exercise, thigh muscle ATP levels were reduced by 21 percent. Much of this loss is attributed to the loss of metabolic end products washed into the bloodstream and lost from the cell. These researchers concluded, "These data indicate that muscle adenine nucleotide loss probably occurs during the very early post exercise period while IMP is elevated and before the cellular energy state is sufficiently recovered to fully reaminate IMP [or restore IMP to AMP]." In other words, they found that the loss of ATP and cellular energy charge occurred as a result of breakdown of AMP and the loss of break down products into the blood.

Additional research by Dr. Terjung has also shown that fast-twitch and slow-twitch muscle fibers differ in their ability to restore lost energy. In this study it was determined that some fast-twitch muscle fibers had a relatively high capacity to restore lost energy and others had a low capacity. Slow twitch fibers were in the middle. It was found that fast-twitch fibers restore energy at the rate of 0.30 percent to 1.06 percent per hour while slow-twitch fibers restore energy at the rate of 0.44 percent to 0.55 percent per hour. If muscles lose 28 percent of their energy charge during exercise, as was found in one study, a simple calculation shows that it may take 26 to 93 hours to fully recover from strenuous exercise! As will be seen below, ribose shortens this recovery time by a wide margin.

Looking at the effect of ribose on recovery of energy charge in different muscle fiber types, Drs. Tullson and Terjung showed dramatic effects. Their research proved that ribose increases the rate of adenine nucleotide restoration in both fast-twitch and slow-twitch muscles by a whopping 3.4 to 4.3 times!

These dramatic results prove that giving ribose increased the ability of both the fast- and slow-twitch muscles of the leg to produce energy-producing compounds and recharge their energy batteries. In addition, these results were constant, whether the muscle was at rest or exercising at high intensity. Using the same math as before, we can now see that these muscle cells could regenerate their energy charge in 6 to 22 hours rather than 26 to 93 hours, as was seen without ribose. In every muscle type tested, ribose improved the ability of the muscle to return to peak performance, fast.

Look again at these results. During exercise, production of ATP, ADP, and AMP slows down. Most energy producing molecules are made while the cell is resting. However, giving ribose allowed muscles to produce more energy molecules even during exercise than untreated muscles produced at rest.

In research that has not yet been published, Dr. Terjung has found that ribose is also effective in keeping these energy molecules in the cell. He has found that ribose will increase the ability of the muscle to save, or salvage, these life-giving molecules by as much as 700 percent! This seems to be convincing evidence that ribose helps both fast- and slow-twitch muscle cells restore energy quickly, allowing the cell to respond to intense and frequent exercise more efficiently and effectively.

At this time there are no direct studies showing how ribose can improve ATP levels in humans during exercise. This type of research is now underway. There is no reason to suspect, however, that the results in man would be any different than those found in test animals. It is reasonable to conclude that ribose administration before, during, and following strenuous exercise will help skeletal muscles regain their energy charge and strength, improve overall performance, and allow rapid energy recovery.

OTHER STUDIES WITH RIBOSE

Ribose is a wondrously effective nutrient. Its affects on heart and muscle cell energy are well researched and clear. Anyone concerned with improving or maintaining energy in their heart or skeletal muscles should include ribose in their nutrition regimen. This is true because ribose is the simplest molecule that is directly related to producing and saving these important life-giving compounds. But what else can ribose do? Is it effective in any other metabolic conditions? The answer, again, is yes.

Thallium-201 Testing

Testing known as Thallium-201 imaging is used by doctors to locate regions of the heart that do not receive enough blood flow or have been damaged by a heart attack or disease. Ribose can help doctors locate these regions before they hurt the heart irreversibly. Several studies have shown this. One study in particular determined that ribose given before and after blood flow to the heart was restricted allowed doctors to locate damaged areas more effectively. Ribose did this by better distributing the Thallium, allowing defective areas to show up better in the test. Additionally, this study showed that giving ribose helped the heart recover function. In fact, without ribose, hearts continued to show a decrease in function 60 minutes following reduced blood flow, while ribose-treated hearts showed marked improvement.

Muscle Soreness

Enzyme deficiencies in muscle may cause rapid loss of ATP and total energy charge. People suffering from these deficiencies have cramping and muscle soreness following even brief, light exercise. Walking across a room may be enough, for example, to cause these severe symptoms, forcing the person to stop and rest before continuing. A significant number of people suffer from these deficiencies in one form or another. It is estimated that about 2 percent of the entire population have these muscle enzyme deficiencies and about 25 percent of these people show moderate to severe symptoms. In the U.S. alone, this could be as many as 1.4 million people or more!

The University of Munich in Germany has been at the forefront of research showing that ribose may be the answer to helping those suffering from these disorders. Several studies have provided convincing evidence of this. One study is particularly significant. A 55-year-old man suffered from painful, exercise-induced long lasting stiffness of his muscles. Throughout his life, he had been a sportsman, performing gymnastic exercises, as well as walking, cycling, or skiing in the mountains. These activities had to be stopped when he started to develop severe pain and stiffness in his arms and legs during exercise. It took several days for the pain to cease between exercise bouts and finally he had to stop altogether. Soon after this patient began taking ribose, the symptoms stopped and the patient was able to return to normal activity.

Ribose may not produce these results in every subject. However, there have been several reports as to the effectiveness of ribose in reducing these symptoms. Muscle soreness and cramping is directly related to energy charge in people with these disorders. Again, it is clear that ribose has the effect of increasing cellular energy levels so that routine exercise can continue without distress.

Diabetes

It is critically important for diabetics to control the level of glucose in their blood. Insulin is the hormone that is normally produced by the body to keep glucose levels in check. Diabetic patients, however, are not able to produce enough insulin to control glucose levels and they may rise to critical levels if the glucose is not controlled by other means. Generally, insulin is given by infusion to keep glucose levels in check. Ribose has been shown to increase the rate of insulin production in both animals and humans.

The positive effects of ribose on controlling glucose levels in diabetics have not been studied extensively. However, one researcher concluded, "Since ribose can be utilized by the diabetic, does not contribute to hyperglycemia [or high blood glucose levels] and limits fat mobilization, further investigation of the possible beneficial effect of administration of this sugar in uncontrolled diabetes is warranted." No such follow up studies have been reported to show this benefit conclusively, but it is possible that ribose may provide such a benefit to diabetics in the future.

Now that you know all about the benefits of ribose, the next chapter will explain how much to take, when to take it, and more.

7
USING RIBOSE

Research on ribose has been going on for several years. However, up until now the manufacturing processes for making ribose were so expensive that it was out of reach to consumers. A process has now been developed, however, that is able to make this important nutrient available. Like other supplements—creatine, pyruvate, and L-carnitine for example—a manufacturing process needed to be found before the supplements could be sold economically. Recent advances in biotechnology have made all these possible. This ribose technology may be the most important recent find in producing a product really capable of maintaining or increasing energy stores in the heart and muscle cells following restricted circulation or intense exercise.

WHO SHOULD TAKE RIBOSE?

Everyone concerned about his or her cardiovascular health can benefit from ribose. However, the degree to which they may benefit is difficult to determine. Certainly, anyone with diminished blood flow to the heart or skeletal muscle would be a prime candidate for ribose supplementation. Those suffering with muscle enzyme deficiencies may also show improvement with ribose. However, whether non-athletes or weekend athletes will gain a dramatic benefit is questionable.

Weekend athletes who have the entire week to restore their muscle energy charge between exercise bouts may not need ribose to recover cellular energy levels. Those exercising to exhaustion frequently during the week, however, may benefit. Three or four exercise bouts per week may not provide enough time between sessions for energy levels to return to normal. One day of rest between heavy exercise bouts will probably not be sufficient to fully restore energy charge in muscle. There is clear and convincing evidence in humans to show that this is true.

Certainly serious athletes can benefit. Ribose should be particularly effective in intense exercise requiring short bursts of supramaximal activity. These sports may include sprinting, basketball, hockey, weightlifting, power lifting, volleyball, soccer, and tennis. Participating in these sports only occasionally may not require ribose supplementation.

HOW MUCH TO TAKE AND WHEN TO TAKE IT

To keep cellular ATP levels at their highest, ribose should be taken every day. Maintenance doses of 3 to 5 grams per day should be enough to maintain normal ATP levels. If you are a serious competitor, or are concerned about your cardiovascular health, you may want to take more. In this case 5 to 10 grams per day may be needed. However, you should try the lower doses first and move up if you think it is necessary. For those suffering from muscular enzyme deficiencies, a little more may be needed. Dr. Manfred Gross at the University of Munich has reported in a published article that 4 to 10 grams per day, taken about one-half to 1 hour before exercise, and then supplementing with another 4-gram dose during strenuous exercise worked in the MADD patient discussed earlier in this booklet.

The research is clear on one point, however. Taking ribose both before and after ischemia or strenuous exercise will increase the benefit. Your heart and muscle cells need a little time to build up the pools of ribose-containing compounds *before* oxidative stress to assure best performance. If your muscles become sore or cramped after even mild exercise, you may want to modify the dose regimen. Try taking 10 grams of ribose before beginning any physical exercise and then supplementing with additional doses of 4 grams every 30 minutes during and at the conclusion of exercise. If this works, the amount of ribose taken can be cut back until the proper individual dose level has been found.

Choosing ribose supplements is fairly easy, as one supplement is not any better than another, with the exception of choosing a reputable manufacturer that works under strict, controlled conditions, using sound production practices. The purity of supplements should always be taken into consideration.

Ribose can be taken as a drink, chewable tablet, capsule, energy bar or any other form. It is practically tasteless, but is slightly sweet. Ribose should not be taken with protein drinks, however, because the ribose may react with the amino acids in the protein and lose effectiveness in the body.

RIBOSE WITH OTHER ENERGY SUPPLEMENTS

Ribose may actually enhance the effect of these other supplements. Here's an example: Use of creatine as a supplement to increase muscle cell energy has grown dramatically in recent years. Creatine is the molecule used by muscle cells to recycle ADP to ATP to help keep energy levels high during intense, strenuous exercise. Even with creatine supplementation, however, energy-producing molecules are degraded during exercise and lost from the cell. If these substrate molecules are lost, they are of no further value to creatine. No amount of creatine in the cell can replace them. Consequently, total energy charge and the size of the ATP pool decreases. No matter how much supplemental creatine is taken, this metabolic process cannot be totally avoided. Ribose is effective in helping to save and rebuild these energy-producing substrate molecules. Working in combination, ribose and creatine may produce a benefit that exceeds that of creatine alone. No scientific research has been conducted to show this directly, but the biochemical evidence is clear. The presence of available substrate molecules is of prime importance in maintaining and restoring energy to muscle cells during strenuous exercise. Ribose can be the missing link.

The same thing is true for L-carnitine, pyruvate, pyruvate/creatine combinations, or other energy supplements. While these compounds may work on their own, their effectiveness is diminished as your heart and skeletal muscles lose those all important ATP substrates. Loss of substrate molecules means that these supplements cannot perform the work of rebuilding ATP levels in muscle cells. Ribose helps the heart and skeletal muscles save or restore these substrates. Increased substrate availability is key to maintaining peak energy charge and heart and muscle function.

IS IT SAFE?

Ribose is found naturally in all the cells of the body. In fact, it is found in all the cells of every living creature, plant or animal. It is safe, effective, and is the simplest molecule in the important reactions aimed at building or restoring energy in all the cells of the body. The effectiveness of ribose in energy metabolism is particularly important in the heart and skeletal muscles where the natural pathways to energy production are slow.

Research has shown that up to 60 grams of ribose per day may be taken without even light complications. At such high doses, though, some people have experienced diarrhea and slight decreases in blood glucose levels. It is suggested, however, that you stick to levels less than 20 grams per day. At these levels, you should experience no side effects at all. Again, it must be emphasized that long-term studies on high doses of ribose administration have not been done. However, there is no biochemical reason to think that they would be harmful. Excess ribose is passed easily through the urine.

You have seen how and why ribose works. This natural, safe compund can truly be called the supreme energy source.

CONCLUSION

By now, you should have enough information to know if ribose supplementation is for you. In the end, you must be the judge. If you are a serious competitor, a hard-charging weekend athlete, have decreased blood flow to your heart or extremities, have muscle enzyme deficiencies, or are just concerned about your cardiovascular health, ribose may help. In all of these situations the heart and skeletal muscles use energy faster than it can be replaced. Ribose is effective in rebuilding these critical energy stores, keeping the heart and skeletal muscles at their peak.

No one can say that taking ribose will help everyone or make him or her feel more energetic. Nor can anyone say that athletic performance will improve for all individuals. The scientific evidence is clear, however, that ribose will help heart and skeletal muscle cells maintain their energy charge and normal function and that taking ribose before, during, and after periods of high-intensity exercise or restricted blood flow increases its effectiveness.

Ribose is a wondrously effective nutrient. It is simple and safe, natural and effective. Ribose is nature's way of increasing energy and maintaining normal function of the heart and skeletal muscles. Ribose is the key ingredient to keeping energy levels high and performance at its peak—and in today's fast-paced world, don't we all need to keep our energy levels at their peak?

GLOSSARY

Aerobic metabolism. Metabolism in the cell that takes place in the presence of oxygen.

Adenine nucleotides. Compounds containing ribose, adenine, and one to three phosphate molecules. ATP, ADP, and AMP are all adenine nucleotides. These compounds provide energy to all living cells.

Anaerobic metabolism. Metabolism in the cell that takes place when there is not sufficient oxygen supplied by the blood to maintain aerobic metabolism.

ATP (adenosine triphosphate). An adenine nucleotide containing three phosphate molecules. ATP is the prime source of energy for all living cells. It produces energy when the chemical bond holding one of the phosphate molecules is broken from the ATP molecule forming ADP, inorganic phosphate and energy.

ADP (adenosine diphosphate). An adenine nucleotide containing two phosphate molecules. ADP is formed from ATP when one of the phosphate molecules are removed for energy production in the cell.

AMP (adenosine monophosphate). An adenine nucleotide containing one phosphate molecule. AMP is formed when one of the phosphate molecules from ADP is broken off.

Anoxia. A condition in which there is insufficient oxygen supplied to the cell to maintain aerobic metabolism.

Creatine monohydrate. A compound found in the mitochondria of heart and skeletal muscle cells used by the cell to accept inorganic phosphate molecules split from ATP and awaiting reattachment to ADP.

Glossary

Creatine phosphate. A compound formed when the inorganic phosphate separated from ATP during energy production attaches to creatine monohydrate.

De novo. A Latin term meaning "new." In biochemical terms, *de novo* synthesis refers to the cell's ability to form new compounds. As used here, *de novo* describes the metabolic process through which the cell produces new energy-producing compounds.

Deoxyribonucleic acid (DNA). DNA is the genetic material found in all living cells. This material passes the genetic code from one generation to the next.

DNA. See Deoxyribonucleic acid.

Enzymes. Enzymes are proteins that cause certain biochemical reactions to occur. They are very specific. Certain enzymes produce only those functions they are designed to perform. Enzymes are absolutely necessary for normal function of cellular metabolism.

Fast-twitch muscle fiber (FT). Fast-twitch skeletal muscle fibers are recruited to contract during moderate- to high-intensity exercise to produce brief but powerful contractions.

5-phosphoribosyl-1-pyrophosphate (PRPP). Formed by adding phosphate molecules to ribose. This compound is the starting point for the production of energy-producing compounds in the heart and skeletal muscles.

Glucose. A six carbon sugar (therefore a carbohydrate) that is the starting point for many metabolic reactions in the body.

Glucose-6-phosphate dehydrogenase (G-6-PDH). An enzyme found in the metabolic pathway from glucose to ribose.

Glycogen. A chain of glucose molecules. Glycogen is used by the body to store glucose for energy production.

IMP (Inosine monophosphate). A compound used by skeletal muscle cells (particularly red fast-twitch cells) to store energy-producing compounds so they are not washed out of the cell. IMP is formed from AMP.

Ischemia. A term referring to a restriction in blood flow to an organ (including the heart or skeletal muscles). In ischemic conditions, the cells are not able to get enough oxygen from the blood to maintain normal aerobic metabolism.

Mitochondria. A sub-unit of a cell (including heart and skeletal muscle cells) in which energy is produced.

Myoadenylate deaminase deficiency disease (MADD). A muscle enzyme deficiency disease in which sufferers are unable to adequately recycle energy. As ATP is used, the break down products are quickly lost from the cell. As a result, these patients have severe muscle soreness and cramping that significantly restricts their physical activities.

Myokinase reaction. The reaction in which ATP is formed by combining two ADP to form one ATP and one AMP. The myokinase reaction is called upon by skeletal muscle in high-intensity exercise when anaerobic metabolism occurs.

Pyruvate. A 3-carbon compound used to produce energy. Pyruvate can be formed from either glucose or ribose (as well as other compounds).

Ribonucleic acid (RNA). A genetic compound containing ribose. In animal cells, RNA is used to pass the genetic information used to produce proteins. In the cell, RNA is used to constantly maintain adequate levels of proteins, including enzymes.

Ribose. A naturally occurring five carbon (pentose) sugar found in all living cells. Ribose is the compound used by the heart and skeletal muscle cells to produce PRPP, which is required for salvage and *de novo* production of energy-producing compounds, or adenine nucleotides. Ribose is formed naturally in the heart and skeletal muscles from glucose through a series of slow and energy consuming biochemical reactions.

RNA. See Ribonucleic acid.

Slow-twitch muscle fiber (ST). As opposed to fast-twitch fibers, slow-twitch fibers are called upon for slower muscular contractions, such as those in standing, walking, or jogging.

SELECTED REFERENCES

Alexander R, Schlant R, Fuster V, eds. *The Heart.* McGraw-Hill, New York, 1998.

Angello D, Wilson R, Gee D. "Effect of Ribose on Thallium-201 Myocardial Redistribution." *Journal of Nuclear Medicine* 29: 1943–1950, 1988.

Angello D, Wilson R, Gee D, Perlmutter N. "Recovery of Myocardial Function and Thallium 201 Redistribution Using Ribose." *American Journal of Cardiac Imaging* 3(4): 256–265, 1989.

Asimakis G, Zwischenberger J, Inners-McBride K, Sordahl L, Conti V. "Postischemic Recovery of Mitochondrial Adenine Nucleotides in the Heart." *Circulation* 85(6): 2212–2220, 1992.

Barnard R, MacAlpin R, Kattus A, Buckberg G. "Ischemic Response to Sudden Strenuous Exercise in Healthy Men." *Circulation* 48: 936–942, 1973.

Bierman E, Baker E, Plough I, Hall W. "Metabolism of D-Ribose in Diabetes Mellitus." *Diabetes* 8(6): 455–458, 1959.

Chatham J, Challiss R, Radda G, Seymour A-M. "Studies of the protective effect of ribose in myocardial ischaemia by using 31P-nuclear-magnetic-resonance spectroscopy." *Biochemical Society Transactions* 13: 885–886, 1985.

Einzig S, St. Cyr J, Bianco R, Schneider J, Lorenz E, Foker J. Myocardial ATP "Repletion with Ribose Infusion." *Journal of Pediatric Research* 19(4): 127A, 1985.

Ginsberg J, Boucher B, Beaconsfield P. "Hormonal Changes During Ribose-enduced Hypoglycemia." *Diabetes* 19: 23–27, 1970.

Goetz F, Maney J, Greenberg B. "The regulation of insulin secretion: Effects of the infusion of glucose, ribose, and other sugars into the portal veins of dogs." *Journal of Laboratoty and Clinical Medicine* 69(4): 537–557, 1967.

Goodman C, Goetz F. "Oral and Intravenous D-Ribose and Plasma Insulin in Healthy Humans: Effects of Route of Administration and of Epinephrine and Propranolol." *Metabolism* 19(12): 1094–1103, 1970.

Gross M, Reiter S, Zollner N. "Metabolism of D-Ribose Administered Continuously to Healthy Persons and to Patients with Myoadenylate Deaminase Deficiency." *Klinische Wochenschrift* 67: 1205–1213, 1989.

Gross M, Kormann R, Zollner N. "Ribose Administration during Exercise: Effects on

Substrates and Products of Energy Metabolism in Healthy Subjects and a Patient with Myoadenylate Deaminase Deficiency." *Klinische Wochenschrift* 69: 151–155, 1991.

Gross M, Zollner N. " Serum Levels of Glucose, Insulin, Klinische Wochenschrift 69: 31–36, 1991.

Halter J, Schwartz M, Goetz F. "The Effect of Oral and Intravenous D-Ribose on Plasma Insulin Levels in Unanesthetized Dogs." *Proceedings of the Society of Experimental Biological Medicine* 127(4): 1147–1151, 1968.

Hellsten-Westling Y, Norman B, Balsom P Sjodin B. "Decreased resting levels of adenine nucleotides in human skeletal muscle after high-intensity training." *Journal of Applied Physiology* 74(5): 2523–2528, 1993.

Lee H, Graeff R, Walseth T. "Cyclic ADP-ribose and its metabolic enzymes." *Biochemie* 77: 345–355, 1995.

Martinz-Augustin O, Boza J, Navarro J, Martinez-Valverde A, Araya M, Gil A. "Dietary Nucleotides May Influence the Humoral Immunityin Immunocompromised Children." *Nutrition* 13(5): 465–469, 1997.

Mauser M, Hoffmeister H, Nienaber C, Schaper W. "Influence of Ribose, Adenosine, and "AICAR" on the Rate of Myocardial Adenosine Triphosphate Synthesis during Reperfusion after Coronary Artery Occlusion in the Dog." *Circulation Research* 56(2): 220–229, 1985.

Page T, Yu A, Fontanesi J, Nyhan W. "Developmental disorder associated with increased cellular nucleotidase activity." *Proceedings of the National Academy of Science* 94: 11601–11606, 1997.

Pasque M, Spray T, Pellom G, Van Trigt P, Peyton R, Currie W, Wechsler A. "Ribose-enhanced myocardial recovery following ischemia in the isolated working rat heart." *Journal of Thoracic and Cardiovascular Research* 83: 390–398, 1982.

Pasque M, Wechsler A. " Metabolic Intervention to Affect Myocardial Recovery Following Ischemia." *Annals of Surgery* 200(1): 1–10, 1984.

Patten B. "Beneficial Effect of D-Ribose in Patient with Myoadenylate Deaminase Deficiency." *Lancet* May 8:1071, 1982.

Perlmutter N, Wilson R, Angello D, Palac R, Lin J, Brown B. "Ribose Facilitates Thallium-201 Redistribution in Patients with Coronary Artery Disease." *Journal of Nuclear Medicine* 32: 193–200, 1991.

Pliml W, von Arnim T, Stablein A, Hofmann H, Zimmer H-G, Erdmann E. "Effects of ribose on exercise-induced ischaemia in stable coronary artery disease." *Lancet* 340: 507–510, 1992.

Reibel D, Rovetto M. "Myocardial ATP synthesis and mechanical function following oxygen deficiency." *American Journal of Physiology* 234(5): H620-H624, 1978.

St. Cyr J, Bianco R, Schneider J, Mahoney J, Tveter K, Einzig S, Foker J. "Enhanced High Energy Phosphate Recovery with Ribose Infusion after Global Myocardial Ischemia in a Canine Model." *Journal of Surgical Research* 46: 157–162, 1989.

Segal S, Foley J. "The Metabolism of D-Ribose in Man." *Journal of Clinical Investigation* 37: 719–735, 1958.

Shin-Ichi K, Martin R, Sato R. "Alterations in ATP-sensitive potassium channel sensitivity to ATP in failing human hearts." *American Journal of Physiology* 272: H1656–H1665, 1997.

Stathis C, Febbraio M, Carey M, Snow R. "Influence of sprint training on human skeletal muscle purine nucleotide metabolism." *Journal of Applied Physiology* 76(4): 1802–1809, 1994.

Steele I, Patterson V, Nicholls D. "A Double Blind, Placebo Controlled, Crossover Trial of D-Ribose in McArdleís Disease." *Journal of Neurological Science* 136: 174–177, 1996.

Tullson P, Whitlock D, Terjung R. "Adenine nucleotide degradation in slow-twitch red muscle." *American Journal of Physiology* 258: C258-C265, 1990.

Tullson P, Terjung R. "Adenine nucleotide synthesis in exercising and endurance-trained skeletal muscle." *American Journal of Physiology* 261: C342-C347, 1991.

Tullson P, Bangsbo J, Hellsten Y, Richter E. "IMP metabolism in human skeletal muscle after exhaustive exercise." *Journal of Applied Physiology* 78(1): 146–152, 1995.

Tullson P, Arabadjis P, Rundell K, Terjung R. " IMP reamination to AMP in rat skeletal muscle fiber types." *American Journal of Physiology* 270: C1067-C1074, 1996.

Vance R. West Virginia University. Unpublished data on file.

Wagner D, Gresser U, Zollner N. "Effects of Oral Ribose on Muscle Metabolism during Bicycle Ergometer in AMPD-Deficient Patients." *Annals of Nutritional Metabolism* 35: 297–302, 1991.

Ward H, St. Cyr J, Cogordan J, Alyono D, Bianco R, Kriett J, Foker J. "Recovery of adenine nucleotide levels after global myocardial ischemia in dogs." *Surgery* 96(2): 248–255, 1984.

Whitlock D, Terjung R. "ATP depletion in slow-twitch red muscle of rat." *American Journal of Physiology* 253: C426-C432, 1987.

Wilson R, Palac R. "Ribose accelerates Thallium-201 Redistribution in Patients with Coronary Artery Disease: A Randomized Placebo-Controlled Crossover Trial." *Proceedings of the Society of Nuclear Medicine* 29(5): 953, 1988.

Zimmer H-G, Suchner H, Schad H. " Ribose Intervention in the Cardiac Pentose Phosphate Pathway Is Not Species Specific." *Science* 223: 712–714, 1984.

Zimmer H-G, Ibel H. "Ribose Accelerates the Repletion of the ATP Pool During Recovery from Reversible Ischemia of the Rat Myocardium." *Journal of Molecular and Cellular Cardiology* 16: 863–866, 1984.

Zimmer H-G. "Significance of the 5-Phosphoribosyl-1-Pyrophosphate Pool for Cardiac Purine and Pyrimidine Nucleotide Synthesis: Studies with Ribose, Adenine, Inosine, and Orotic Acid in Rats." *Cardiovascular Drugs and Therapy* 12:179–187, 1998.

Zimmer H-G. "Restitution of myocardial adenine nucleotides: acceleration by administration of ribose." *Journal of Physiology,* Paris 76: 769–775, 1980.

Zimmer H-G, Martius P, Marschner G. "Myocardial infarction in rats: effects of metabolic and pharmacologic interventions." *Basic Research in Cardiology* 84:332–343, 1989.

Zollner N, Reiter S, Gross M, Pongratz D, Reimers C, Gerbitz K, Paetzke I, Duefel T, Hubner G. "Myoadenylate Deaminase Deficiency: Successful Symptomatic Therapy by High Dose Oral Administration of Ribose." *Klinische Wochenschrift* 64: 1281–1290, 1986.

INDEX

Adenine nucleotides. *See* Adenine diphosphate; Adenine monophosphate; Adenine triphosphate; Nucleotides.
Adenosine, 6
Adenosine diphosphate (ADP), 2, 6, 14, 17, 21, 30
   myokinase reaction and, 7–8
Adenosine monophosphate (AMP), 2, 15, 16, 17, 21, 29, 30
   myokinase reaction and, 7–8
Adenosine triphosphate (ATP)
   about, 1–2
   exercise and, 17–19
   muscles and, 5, 14, 15
   myokinase reaction and, 7–8
   production of, 5–8
   ribose and, 9–10, 21, 22, 27, 29
ADP. *See* Adenosine diphosphate.
Aerobic metabolism, 6
AMP. *See* Adenosine monophosphate.
Anaerobic metabolism, 6
Anoxia, 15, 27
Athletes, ribose and, 33–34
ATP. *See* Adenosine triphosphate.

Blood flow, insufficient. *See* Ischemia.

Chatham, John, 28
Circulation, poor, 19–20, 26–28
Creatine phosphate (CrP), 6–7, 14
Creatine supplementation, 35
CrP. *See* Creatine phosphate.

De novo metabolic pathways, 22
Deoxyribonucleic acid (DNA), 9, 11
Diabetes, ribose and, 32
DNA. *See* Deoxyribonucleic acid.
D-ribose. *See* Ribose.

Energy loss
   circulation and, 19–20
   preventing, 20
   replacing, 21–22
Energy production, 6, 7
Exercise, ATP and, 10, 17–19

Fast-twitch muscle fibers (FT), 13–14, 30
5-phosphoribosyl-l-pyrophosphate (PRPP), 22
FT fibers. *See* Fast-twitch muscle fibers.

Glucose, 10, 22–23
Glucose-6-phosphate dehydrogenase (G-6-PDH), 23

Gross, Manfred, 34
G-6-PDH. *See* Glucose-6-phosphate dehydrogenase.

Heart
   energy loss and, 19–20
   ribose and, 26–28, 31
Heart muscle, 15

IMP. *See* Inosine monophosphate.
Inorganic phosphate (Pi), 6
Inosine monophosphate (IMP), 29
Insulin, 32
Involuntary muscle. *See* Smooth muscle.
Ischemia, 10, 15, 17, 19

L-carnitine, 35

MADD. *See* Myoadenylate deaminase deficiency.
Muscle cells, 7, 8
Muscle contraction, ATP and, 5
Muscle soreness, ribose and, 31–32
Muscles, about, 12–13. *See also* Heart muscle; Skeletal muscle.
Myoadenylate deaminase deficiency (MADD), 16
Myokinase reaction, the, 7–8

Nucleic acid. *See* Deoxyribonucleic acid; Ribonucleic acid.
Nucleotides, 10–11, 16

Pi. *See* Inorganic phosphate.
Pliml, Wolfgang, 28
Poor circulation. *See* Circulation, poor.
PRPP. *See* 5-phosphoribosyl-1-pyrophosphate.
Pyruvate, 10, 35

Riboflavin, 11
Ribonucleic acid (RNA), 9, 11
Ribose
   about, 9–10
   athletes and, 33–34
   ATP and, 9–10, 21, 22, 27, 29
   body's use of, 10–11
   dosage, suggested, 34, 35
   heart and, 26–28
   research on, 23–25, 26–32
   safety of, 35–36
   skeletal muscle and, 13, 14, 29–31
   supplementation, 2–3, 11, 23
   supplements, other, and, 35
   who should take it, 33–34
RNA. *See* Ribonucleic acid.

Salvage pathway, 21
Skeletal muscles, 13–14, 16
   ribose and, 29–31
Slow-twitch muscle fibers (ST), 14, 30
Smooth muscle, 12
ST fibers. *See* Slow-twitch muscle fibers.
Stathis, C, 19
Striated muscle, 12–13
Substrate molecules, 14, 35

Terjung, Ronald, 29, 30
Thalium-201 testing, ribose and, 31
Tullson, P., 43

Vance, Robert, 27
Voluntary muscle. *See* Striated muscle.

Ward, Herbert, 20

Zimmer, Heinz-Gerd, 20